Introduction

Why don't we know?

So where are the answers?

Brain Fog

Menopause Journey

New Beginnings with Brain Fog

Me Time

Tired? I am Exhausted!

Are you hot or is it me?

Oooops!

Palpitations

Weight

Sleep

Moody

Ouch!

Fun

Periods

What are you eating?

Don't forget to stretch!

GW00456453

Intuitive Living

Prescribed Drugs (from your doctor)

General Day to Day

Conclusion

References

After Thought

INTRODUCTION

Hi my name is Kim.

What do you need to know about me?

I have no idea really, I am 47 at the time of writing this book, with a Birthday at the weekend.

I am happily married, to my second husband and together we have six wonderful children.

After much thought, discussion and planning we relocated to live in North Cyprus, yes the bit thats not recognised by the rest of the world but is absolutely the place that makes us the happiest!

It goes without saying that of course we miss the children and our family and friends but still this was the right move for us now.

I am currently sitting on the upstairs balcony, I can see the sea and the mountains and all around me are fields with the sound of nature, what better place for inspiration.

So I have decided to write down my Menopausal Journey, I had been thinking about it for the best part of a year and then thought that's it just start writing and see how it goes. I just want all women to have some knowledge of what is coming from a normal perspective.

This is a very personal account of what I am living with and through and how I am learning and sharing so that hopefully you will feel normal too.

I also feel that I should say a massive THANK YOU to my husband, who lets face it is also living this with me!

Now I want to give you a little insight into how I am writing this book, I have never written a book before and I am sure there are all sorts of rules you are supposed to follow, however, I am just writing. One of the big things because of my amazing brain function or lack of it some days (you will understand soon) I do find that I go back and reread what I have written frequently but I didn't want to correct myself or change, but rather be honest and add as I go as this is a record of my journey and life isn't all straight lines, I hope that makes sense as you read it and you understand the thinking behind it. To be honest I feel like we are just having a chat over a cuppa.

At the back of this book I will reference all the books and articles, podcasts and accounts on Instagram and Facebook that I have either referred to in this book or that I have felt useful during my journey.

CHAPTER 1

WHY DON'T WE KNOW?

We are taught so much at school, however, we still aren't teaching life skills, we may all be able to breakdown the text of a popular Shakespeare play or know what X and Y equal but we don't teach anything about actual life!

Now maybe you are shouting at me while reading this, telling me that this is the parents role, but who teaches the parents?

But I digress, the what that they don't teach us, the us being women, is Menopause.

Considering the massive impact that this has on our lives it's surprising that here we are in 2019 and its still a whispered conversation. Now this is beginning to change but only if you are interested and actually go looking for the information.

Am I an expert, do I have any qualifications in this subject?

Well the answer is no, however, I am a woman and I am living through it so I think I have an opinion and an experience that could help others.

This book is really my journey through the minefield that is Menopause, how I cope, what I have discovered and if it helps one person with their journey well thats amazing!

CHAPTER 2

SO WHERE ARE THE ANSWERS?

So how do we find out the answers to our questions?

Well this is a very good question and one that I am still struggling with.

First stop I guess should be your doctor, I mean thats what we do if we have worrying symptoms, they have the knowledge right?

For me though, I knew that if I went to the doctors there would be a strong possibility that he would want to put me on HRT (Hormone Replacement Therapy) but that for me is really not an option. Everyone is different of course but as I say for me this option just isn't right.

So I spoke to lots of people I know who are around my age or older and asked them, you know, I feel like this, have/ do you? Slowly I began to realise that most people in my age bracket were feeling and going through things very similar to me they just weren't necessarily chatting about it.

Next I took to the internet, it really is a wonderful resource and there are people (woman mainly, I haven't come across a man yet but I am sure there is one) who want to tell you about Menopause and help you but you do really have to look and search them out.

I have found some great Facebook pages, not all helpful, Instagram Accounts and there is some literature out there too but the thing that shocked me the most is that there really isn't very much and as I said you have to go find it.

So here we are……………………….

CHAPTER 3

BRAIN FOG

Lets go back a bit not far, just three years, I think this is when I started to notice changes. Actually, I have just read that back, its about 5 or 6 years! At first it was funny, things that we would laugh about at work but then it became more distressing and actually when I look back now quite scary.

Let me paint the picture for you.

I was working full time, my hubby was also working full time and like most people living in the UK we were working huge amounts of hours and so were really continuously tired. We also have children, who bring there own challenges, this is not about them and actually only one of them was living at home with us at the time.

So there we are working our little hearts out and then some days I would find that I was being a little forgetful. Not a huge drama, I would just make sure that I always had my note pad with me and record everything and I mean everything. Times, places, jobs that needed to be completed, peoples names, instructions on how to do things, passwords. I am sure there was more but I forget!

When this happened I would laugh, make light of the situation. "Menopause moment!"

But actually it was getting worse.

The harder I worked, the more responsibility I took on, the more pressure I put myself under the worse the forgetfulness became. It was like a fog that got into my brain so I couldn't see.

It got so bad at one point that I regularly used to have to wake my son up to unlock my phone because I just couldn't remember the password for my work phone. Annoyingly, this had to change frequently which is perfectly sensible, it was a work phone, but so unhelpful for me. I felt like I was going mad. I do remember at one point sitting down with my husband to explain to him about this brain fog as I was becoming extremely frustrated by it. "Did he think I had Alzheimer's?"

We noticed that when we had a holiday and some the stress wasn't there that the fog began to clear so we knew it was not Alzheimers, but what was it? I had friends of differing ages and some of them were having Menopause symptoms but none of them had the fog. Most had hot flushes in the day at various times but I didn't have these.

In the back of my head I remembered mum having menopause symptoms, I remember her saying something like "there are 20 symptoms and I have all 20" but I didn't remember her ever mentioning the fog. Hardly surprising I guess!!

So what's the fog?

How can I explain it?

Well, a typical day when it was at its worse, I would wake up and then have to think really hard what day is it. Is it a work day? Where was I supposed to be today?

At the time my role was similar to an area manager, some days I would work from home or I could be travelling to a client meeting or in a unit supporting staff. It was important I knew where I was going to be.

Even this task, which we all do everyday without thinking was a huge problem, my brain would just be blank. It was like someone had switched the light off at the end of the previous day and had forgotten to turn it back on again.

The analogy I have used to explain this fog is to use my husband as an example he is all about numbers, a human calculator if you please, give him a sum he sees it in this mind and gives you the answer. My thing is English, can't spell a word, I can see it in my mind and spell if for you. This is the bit of my brain that had been switched off. It was an empty nothingness.

Somedays this would last all day, somedays once I got going it would improve and somedays I was functioning fine.

Now this is scary, why was it happening and how the hell could I overcome it and why didn't other people suffer with this?

I know now that they do, but I haven't know that for very long and I have to add, not everyone has this symptom during their Menopause journey.

Actually finding out that this is a normal symptom really helped me to manage the fog and probably because I stopped worrying about it so much it eased.

(As I said at the beginning of this book, if I can help one person then I am happy, if I had been able to read something like this at the beginning of this interesting journey I think it would have relieved a lot of anxiety, I will not be apologising for repeating this statement often.)

So now I have been retired for nearly two years and I still have the brain fog but I am a much more chilled relaxed person now. Due to the life that we live there is no daily pressure, its absolutely fine if I need to have a slow day, no one cares and my husband is ace at understanding what I am going about .

CHAPTER 3 1/2

Menopause Journey

I just have to interrupt myself here to explain why I am going to continually call this a menopause journey.

I came across this information about 6 months ago and I have to say it was a bit of an eye opener so I suggest you go put the kettle on for a cup of tea, sit in your most comfy chair, with a blanket and a biscuit if it feels right, before reading the next bit.

Ready.....

Okay Menopause is actually this;

2-8 years of peri menopause * *** - your body beginning to change and dry up, in one of my sons most eloquent descriptions!

1 Day Menopause - the birthday celebration of 1 year of no periods!

the rest of your life post menopause

Are you okay? I know its a bit of a revelation isn't it. I naively thought that I would have Menopause (hot flushes) for a few years and then off I would go with the rest of my life.

Apparently not!!

Basically, we as women are going to go through a journey of ailments, the last book I read said there are 220 different symptoms, obviously we are not all going to have all of them. Gosh, could you image that! Let's not. Some of us might just have a few, others more and some will pass and then we might get new ones and some will just stay with us like a faithful companion.

Are you excited now for your journey?

Now I don't want to cause any alarm or sadness but we do need the facts so we can cope and get on living. I remember feeling quite down and low about how I was going to manage and then I had a bit of a lightbulb moment and thought, you know what this isn't a disease it just part of life and so it is not going to beat me.

*** everyone of us is completely different so this could be a different length of time, shorter or longer. In the same way the onset of this is a different age for all of us.

Lets just take a moment to let one of those statements really sink in;

This is not a disease.

CHAPTER 4

NEW BEGINNINGS
WITH BRAIN FOG

So we need some positivity now after that bombshell!

The brain fog has eased, I don't think I would be able to sit here and write this if it hadn't, so thank goodness for that.

Now that I am retired, yes I retired young! I have more time to listen to my body and discover what makes me worse and what I can do to help with these different symptoms. Now don't get me wrong this doesn't happen overnight and I am still figuring it out, I have been retired for nearly 2 years now.

So firstly, being retired does help!

Not feeling under so much pressure and being able to do normal daily jobs, like going food shopping, once felt like a massive chore that I had a small window of time to complete the task in, I always wrote a list, mostly I forgot the list. Yes, we all do it, get home to realise that the most important thing you needed was still back on the shelf in the shop. Once I had more time I found that my brain began to calm, so I was able to think more clearly, don't get me wrong I still sometimes forget the list and I still sometimes get home without having bought the most important item!

Baby steps remember, celebrate each small positive A food shop that doesn't end in tears, whoop whoop and happy days!

Sometimes these little "moments" can be quite amusing and bring so much laughter a resent moment that I can share is one that I probably will never live down.

We had decided that on the Friday night we would have steak for dinner, I had got the steak out of the freezer ready to defrost, I did think at that time that the steak felt lighter than usual but it was a fleeting thought that came and went. On the Friday I took the steak out of the fridge to reach room temperature ready to cook, then something can't remember what, happened so I popped the steak back into the fridge as I knew I wasn't going to be cooking, saying my hubby that we must eat it the following night. Saturday evening came, steaks came out the fridge so they would be ready to cook, hubby had suggested wedges so they were cooking nicely in the oven, I opened up the wrapping so I could season the steaks BUT oh dear, this was not steak. I closed the wrappings back up, breathed opened it and looked again.

Yep! It was half a lemon drizzle cake!!!!!!!!!!!

I cried, apologised, cried some more then we laughed heartily for quite a while, luckily I have an extremely understanding hubby, once we had stopped laughing he took us out for a curry and a glass of wine.

It still makes me giggle now when I think of it, I mean why didn't I check before but there it is. These things happen and we have to laugh and move on, its not the end of the world and to be honest we could have just had a plate of wedges for dinner and cake for dessert and no harm done.

So what have we established so far, laughter is very important.

This is not a disease but something to embrace and it is important to have ME time.

I will explain a little more in the next chapter about Me Time but I wanted to tell you what else eases my brain fog.

So exercise is a big one, when I was working I did try a few things but because I was always running on empty I wasn't ever consistent but it turns out this really makes a difference. In the last year I have discovered Intuitive Eating which lead me to Intuitive Living and exercise is part of this and it really means in simple terms that rather than exercising because you have to burn calories or because your FitBit/Apple Watch or something similar is shouting at you to complete the daily task that you actually exercise for how it makes you feel.

Now I am not talking about feeling out of breath and sweaty, I am talking about your mental heath and how you actually feel once you get into the exercise and after you have finished. How it can actually set you up to have a good day!

Lets stop for a minute and hold that thought, I am not saying that regular exercise is going to solve all your problems or cure your mental health problems, or make your brain fog disappear but it does help. I have read numerous articles and books about just that but it has taken me awhile to realise that "they" are right. For me if I am consistent with my exercise the brain fog lessens. Happy days!

During the last year I have tried all sorts of different exercises to find out what I actually like because if you had asked me a couple of years ago what I liked I would have laughed. I don't do exercise, I certainly don't like it, enjoy exercise and me are not words that you put in the same sentence. However, this is not correct. I do love some exercise.

I love walking our dogs, swimming in our pool (yes! we have a pool and I am so grateful for that luxury that we have), resistance workouts I am now the proud owner of dumbbells and kettle bells! I also absolutely love YOGA! Why did I not know this before, I now do some sort of yoga practice everyday, sometimes I have been known to get the giggles either because I have tied myself up and then collapsed in a heap or the dogs have tried to help me, laughter is good so who cares. For me the magic part about yoga is that not only is my body becoming stronger and more flexible but it also gives me that Me Time I spoke about earlier, I don't think of anything apart from how I am breathing and moving my body, it fabulous. I am a big fan, can you tell?!

The other thing that I have found that helps the old brain fog to lessen, I discovered completely by accident and that is vitamin B1.

So because we live in North Cyprus as the spring arrives so do the things that bite, mosquitoes! Now last year we managed okay with bug spray and anti histamine but now we have been here a little while we have discovered other techniques used by the locals, like lemon/lime cologne and vitamin B1. We had been told to buy some of these vitamins take them through the summer and within a week the mosquitoes should have 1. stopped biting and 2. any bite you do get will be hardly noticeable. (also, you smell of Marmite for the first couple of days, its fine only you can smell it honest).

So, we take the tablets, after the first week the bites are really non existent and then all of a sudden I realise, I have been talking like a normal person. No missing words, no strange sentences that I just expect my hubby to understand and decipher!

Time to do some research, mostly its B12 that is suggested if you ask Google about help with Menopause but wait, search vitamin B1 and guess what it helps with brain function.

YES, happy dance time, another thing that is helping me to feel "normal".

Now I do have have to add here that although it has made a difference I don't take these all the time, just over the summer mosquito months. Since stopping taking them the fog hasn't rushed back in, yes it is there some days but that okay I know what it is and the people around me know that have this brain fog, so I will tell them that it's not a good word day. They are my friends so they don't care and some day they might be having a bad word day too so you can image the conversations that ensue.

So if I was pushed to answer my own question at the beginning of this chapter, does being retired help? I think I would have to say yes for me, as I have had to travel this experience to find out the information and answers I was looking for but in general I would say no now you can read this book, it should bridge the gap for you and take the pressure off.

CHAPTER 5

ME TIME

Now depending on what age you are, this can be a strange subject. It's definitely a generation thing, not always but mainly the younger you are the more self aware of Me Time you are, in our world of Social Media and self care Sundays etc

I am sure my mum won't mind me telling you that she for one doesn't understand the term Me Time, its just not who she is and there is nothing wrong with that but I have to say the more I have explored this the more I am beginning to understand the benefits of Me Time. Honestly, mum does have me time it's just that she hasn't labelled it.

So what is it, do you have to be retired?

Well the simple answer to that is a big fat NO!

Anyone can have me time but you have to decide what works best for you and how you are going to fit it into your day, without and this I think is the most important detail, **without** feeling guilty.

Yes you have to hold down your job, clean the house, do the washing, feed yourself and your family, in my case run the children about and support them in their learning or clubs etc etc etc I mean the list is completely endless. Even if you are a person without children the call on your time goes on and on and lets remember we all only have a certain amount of hours in the day.

You just have to plan a little bit of time for you, if you can fit in an hour fabulous but to be honest ten minutes everyday would soon start to make a noticeable difference.

So what do we do in Me Time? Below is a list of all the things that came to mind while I was writing this chapter, if I think of anymore I will come back and add the extras, but for now here are some suggestions;

Reading

Meditating

Cooking

Bubble Bath

Shower

Painting your nails

Face Mask

Walking

Having a lay in

Going to bed ten minutes earlier

Watching your favourite TV show (for me The real Housewives of Beverley Hills)

Spending time with friends

Phoning a loved one or friend

Listening to the radio or your favourite music

Going out for dinner

Having a holiday

Cleaning a cupboard out (Yes! Mrs Hinch will confirm a bit of cleaning is good for the soul)

Yoga

Having a cuddle (make sure you know the person you are going to cuddle!)

Laughing

Dancing

Just though of a couple more;

Audio books (I love these but I always fall asleep!)

Podcasts

And a few more that have just popped into my head;

Jigsaw Puzzles

Dot to Dot (Yes, really your mind is thinking about something other than the day)

Colouring (there are some fab adult colouring books out there in the shops at the moment)

Knitting

Crochet

Crosswords

Su Doku

Well, there you go, you can see that some of these things can be fitted into a short space of time but I think mainly Me Time is about stopping, breathing and just giving yourself time to catch yourself up. *It also just occurred to me that the majority of these are free as well.*

Being Mindful is a very popular phrase at the moment but this is really the same principle.

STOP

BREATH

CATCH YOURSELF UP TO NOW

Its amazing how doing one of these things can really help to bring back your focus and still your mind. Now as I said before, I am no expert but I know from having the time to notice that these things have helped me.

If only I had realised a few years ago that rather than collapsing in a heap on the sofa with a glass of red wine planning the next few hours before I went to bed or the tasks for the next day, that I could have gone in the garden watched the clouds, stopped and breathed that just maybe the brain fog would have lessened.

Hindsight is a wonderful thing, but again, that is why I wanted to write this all down, if it helps one person (I won't apologise for repeating this) then I have made a difference and that can ever only be a good thing.

Just recently mum came to stay with us and said that she felt so relaxed and had read so much which she really enjoyed, so now she has gone home to continue taking more time to read. Whether this will continue forever who knows but for now it is giving her the time she needs.

I love reading and always read a little first thing in the morning and usually a little at night before I go to sleep but just recently I have discovered audio books and actually find that these are really relaxing to listen to and help me fall asleep. Quite often I fall asleep before the timer on my chapter has finished and the next night I have to go back a bit, my guilty pleasure just recently has been to have a bath listening to the Archers! I know, but it means that my brain is listening to that so it is quiet, it isn't planning or working at lists etc.

Even though we have retired and can do whatever we want whenever we want I can still find myself thinking, maybe I have been a bit lazy today or I should have done more in the day but the truth is no one actually cares. So I am getting much better at saying to myself, go and take some time to do................... (whatever I feel I need to do). Sometimes it might just be sitting on the balcony watching the sun go down.

CHAPTER 6

Tired? I am Exhausted!

Okay so we have dealt with brain fog, I know that is not going away any time soon, but as you have read I have found a few things that can ease it.

So what else.........................

Being tired, no not just tired, completely and utterly exhausted.

Not just at the end of a day or even just for a day, but a few days maybe a week. I literally could sleep day and night with extra sleep and still feel like I haven't slept for a hundred years. Yes I know that sounds really dramatic but I kid you not that is how it feels.

Saying that I am tired doesn't really describe this symptom very well, there really needs to be another word that sits somewhere between tired and I don't know I can't think how to describe the other end from tired, I had dead come into my head but I think that maybe is being dramatic!

I will describe it for you, when I wake up I know immediately that this is going to be a day where functioning as a human will be hard. My eyes really don't want to be open and will fight my brain command to wake up. Very occasionally ,I will give in and let my body sleep some more but as I said before this isn't a disease and I do know that the extra sleep won't make any difference on one of these days.

I move slowly, oh so slowly, my body feels heavy and everything takes an age and it feels like I am moving through treacle, usually on these days the brain fog is there with a vengeance, which is so helpful, the one day I could probably do with my words is the day that my words are quite frankly gone!

As I said, I have an amazing hubby who just goes with the flow and can recognise the signs as much as I can now, so we will have a 'Oh its one of those days' conversations, not sure I am actually that articulate but he knows what I mean. I try on these days to be kind to myself so I don't fill my days with lots of activities but just go with it, move slowly, exercise in whatever way feels right, Yoga is great on these days and just not put any pressure on myself. Now I know I have the luxury of being retired so it really doesn't matter when a slow day occurs but believe me I had these when I was working too and its not fun, I just did whatever it took to get through the day and then as soon as I got home it would be PJ's on, a cup of tea and bed as soon as I needed too. I have been known to be in bed by 7.30pm.

Now at the moment (it may change again) these 'tired' days usually are just that one day but sometimes it can be the best part of the week. It generally occurs when my body is getting ready to have a period, so even though they are completely erratic these days and quite hard to see a pattern it is a good early warning system that tells me I am due a period in the very near future. When I have the 'tired' days for a week its almost as if my brain forgets whats going on with my body, I will feel tired the words go, I get irritated that I am tired, I try to deny its happening, I start asking myself why do I feel like this, I shouldn't feel this tired at my age, I haven't done enough to feel this tired, there must be something wrong with me, maybe I should make an appointment with the doctor. By the time I ask myself this I get the aha moment, remember this is peri menopause!

Then I calm, remember and within a few days I am back to feeling normal again. This used to happen regularly but in the last few months it has eased, don't get me wrong it hasn't gone but I am getting it for a day in a week, so maybe it will change or maybe I am coming to the end of this symptom.

Either way there is a positive there, so happy dance time!

A fabulous lady that I follow on Instagram shared a post recently that say it was okay to not finish, your best is absolutely good enough, we don't have to be perfect and we don't have to finish that list that we wrote for the day. Once you have this light bulb moment it completely takes the pressure off.

You made the list no one else, no one else cares, so you don't need to either. I know I have already referenced Mrs Hinch but she also acknowledges this point and rather then a To Do list she has a Tadaa list, which is writing down what you have achieved and celebrating that instead.

It really is all about perspective.

Unless you have experienced the complete and total exhaustion it is quite difficult to explain just how tired you feel. Somedays just getting dressed will be the biggest win you have and do you know what, that is okay and its amazing. If only more of us shared this tiredness we wouldn't all be walking about thinking we are the only one going through this. When I was working it was a regular conversation amongst everyone to say that they were tired because the kids had them up in the night or their husbands snoring nearly drove them nuts, but this peri menopausal tired is so much more, I dream of the days I was tired because the kids had worn me out.

I have tried to research this subject but tI haven't found any information out there about how to deal with the "tired", I have come to learn that it is connected to our changing hormones, which of course is the bottom line of this whole journey. I think you could sum up the journey as "Teenagers but in reverse". I mean lets face it quite a few of the symptoms match teenagers, sleeping all day, grumpy, communication skills at zero, walking about in the middle of the night.

Please just remember that you are not on your own, the "tired" is a symptom and is normal and it does pass, well maybe I should say change or lessen as I am still waiting to see if it is going to go completely.

The trouble is in wishing one symptom away is that no sooner has it lessened or gone it gets replaced with something different and that isn't always for the better. I am thinking palpitations (I don't like that one!). There may not be a solution but I have found that if I acknowledge the symptom then it helps.

CHAPTER 7

ARE YOU HOT
OR IS IT ME?

If we are going to talk all things Menopause then we have to have a little chat about hot flushes.

For the most part, remember I don't have any qualification in this field so can't state this as a fact, but it seems to me that every woman going through this journey will experience hot flushes. I am sure that there is an exception to the rule as there always is, so sorry Susan if you don't have them and also hurray for you, go happy dance that one.

Even these though can be different for the individual, just because Susan (sorry if your name is Susan) down the road has mega heat explosions first thing in the morning does not mean that you will.

For me personally, I don't ever get hot flushes during the day, mine are always at night, 9 times out of ten they seem to rev up at 2.00am, and if I drink too much red wine they are worse. There I have said it, some articles may have you believing that red wine can be good for you, certainly if you read The Daily Mail, but in this instance one glass too many and my tropical heatwave is completely out of hand! Also, as a side note one glass too many could be just that one glass, but on another occasion it could be glass number 3 there is no pattern, just another thing to keep me on my toes.

Now remember that we live in a hot country and have two dogs

(I may not have mentioned that before, lets talk about the dogs for a moment, they are two sisters Megan and Tilly about 3 years old, Cyprus Poodles and they like to be everywhere we are and to be honest they are rescue dogs and fought so hard to overcome all their illnesses that we are happy for them to be with us all the time)

So red wine, August night time temperatures, (usually around the 27 degree mark) two dogs you can imagine some nights I am literally lying in a puddle! Sorry that really isn't a pleasant image but that's how it is. To be honest it can also come in handy in the winter when its cold and everyone is complaining about how cold they were, I am happy, I have spent the night with my feet hanging out of the bed very comfortable thank you.

So how many different types of hot flush are there? Well I have no idea but these are the different types that I have encountered observing the people around me.

The standard- it is acknowledged that said hot flush is happening, a period outside with hand flapping maybe required for a short period of time.

The full on waterfall- starts at the feet rises quickly accompanied by bright red skin and by the time its finished the lady in question needs to change her clothes.

The face rain- this is like the waterfall above, apart from the fact that it only affects the face and you have sweat running down your face as if someone has thrown a bucket of water over you.

The delicate flush- barely noticeable, a fan maybe used to cool the said lady gently for a moment before it passes leaving no evidence behind.

The night puddle- you wake up in the middle of the night in a puddle, no more explanation needed.

Now as with everything to do with this subject I am sure there are many scales of each of these descriptions, some better and some worse but please just be aware these are all normal peri menopause moments to be embraced, as lets face it we have to go through it.

It maybe that as you have read these descriptions someone you know at work or socially may come to mind and you will be thinking Ah! so they are going through it too, not everyone wants to shout it from the roof top I guess, but I do think that the more we discuss it and talk about it the more we all understand and the more normal it will become. Also, the men folk amoung us, husbands and sons can understand a little more about what we are going through so it helps them be a little more patient with us.

Hopefully, as you pass Menopause and go into Post Menopause the hot flushes will disappear, I have it on good authority from friends that have already got there that yes they disappear with the very occasional one popping up just to see if you are paying attention.

Just last week I was listening to a podcast where the guest was describing her hot flushes, she described them as having literally the devil bursting our of her chest with all the fire of hell! Well, that's a scenario I haven't come across before and for that I am please. Poor lady I hope she doesn't suffer with hot flushes this intense for too long.

CHAPTER 8

OOOOPS!

Sorry, I just have to interrupt myself here for a minute and share this.

(I wanted this book to be a completely honest and frank view of my journey warts and all (I haven't developed warts yet!))

If you are still drinking your cuppa from earlier I suggest you put it down, I don't want you to spill it down yourself.

Okay, so the hubby and I are off out to do our weekly shop this morning, we collected everything up we needed, said goodbye to the dogs (told them we wouldn't be long, we say that every time no matter the length of our trip out) then off we go to the car. Half way down the drive I stop, laugh and head back to the house.

Hubby is waiting at the gate for me as I head back down the drive to the car, shaking his head enquiring what did I forget was it the list, we had just had a discussion about not forgetting the list.

But oh no, this was much worse or funnier than that,

I hadn't put my flip flops on, Yes you read that right I was off to do the big shop barefoot like a hobbit!!

I ask you.

We will just leave that there I think.

CHAPTER 9

PALPITATIONS

As new symptoms goes this one is not a good one for me, my least favourite if you like, Palpitations, not liking it at all and quite frankly will be glad when it goes. It is a new symptom to me since starting writing this book and I have to say I don't like this one (sorry I already said that, I guess thats how much I really don't like it!) and it's not so easy to laugh off and make light of.

A long time ago, we are talking probably 20 years ago I did suffer from palpitations, at that time I went to the doctors who put me on one of the monitors that you walk around with for 24 hours and then he put me on Beta Blockers, which was awful and I hated them. I didn't stay on them long as they made me feel like a zombie, instead I went to a homeopath, this really helped and the palpitations disappeared. Looking back I know now that these palpitations were due to the immense amount of pressure that I was under, 3 children aged 8 and under and getting a divorce, that would definitely do it!

So now they have started again, I am absolutely not under any type of stress so I knew that this time it was for a different reason. So I Googled, palpitations and the menopause (how did we function before Google?) and jackpot! There it is a symptom.

So what is this like for me, well as with most of the things that affect me they come on at night, usually as I am just going to sleep and it is like a gentle fluttering in my chest, if I concentrate on it and then acknowledge and worry about it, which is completely normal, then it increases and gets worse. I have to have a little chat with myself and calm the situation, I know what this is, there is nothing wrong with my heart, I am not going to die, sounds dramatic but these things run through your head in the middle of the night. Then I yoga breath, in for the count of 5, hold for the count of 5 and breath out slowly for the count of 5. (This technique is actually rather good if you are having trouble sleeping, but thats a whole different chapter)

Usually by the time I get to the end of that I have fallen asleep.

I am aware, through going to counselling myself and through people close to me going to counselling that the brain is clever but also gets distracted or bored depending on how you want to look at it, so palpitations, panic attacks and the like cannot and do not last, usually by the 45 minute mark the boredom for your brain kicks in. I know 45 minutes your thinking thats blooming ages and you are right while you are going through it, 45 minutes can feel like a life time, however once you understand whats happening to you and why, then they don't last this long and you can begin to reduce the time quite successfully.

I also like to say things out loud to my hubby when I am worrying about a pain or a symptom, for me once I have said it and it's out there it usually calms down. I have been know to state in the middle of the night that my palpitations are particular bad this evening. Works wonders for me, then I go back off to sleep, usually leaving my hubby wide awake and unable to go back to sleep. I told you he is a gem.

Please remember that I am sharing my journey and I have listened to my body a lot and I know that this is just another symptom, if you develop something similar it is definite worth checking with your doctor, please always go doctor first.

And let's be honest, I don't know you and I have no idea of your life up until this point so maybe a counselling session is something that you can benefit from to understand your stresses. Even if they are really obvious and right in our faces we don't always notice the why straight away.

Also we don't always connect the dots, I have just been rereading this and did have a little giggle to myself as I was reading that I have no stress now, then I remembered that actually this new symptom that only started recently, it started when my Dad had a heart attack, so clearly that is huge stress, we live in different countries, its my dad (he has made a full recovery by the way).

This event was definitely the trigger to these, however now the stress has passed they have decided to hang around for a while (lets hope not too long).

Update on the palpitations;

Just to update you all on this subject, I have reduced my caffeine intake, coffee related, down from 3 cups a day to 1-2 cups, this is not strict or ridge but I wanted to see if it had an effect, I have also upped my intake of water and tried to get more sleep. These 3 things together seem to be working and the palpitations seem to be no more. So I will keep on with this method and hopefully, everything crossed, they will stay away.

CHAPTER 10

WEIGHT

Right, well now it is time for us to chat about weight. Only if you want to. This is a loaded and difficult subject to approach. I don't want to trigger anyone but I am going to talk, food, diets and feelings. If you want to skip this chapter or visit it a different time, please do. I want this book to help and support you, not to cause you any unnecessary stress.

Maybe we should all go and make another cup of tea, grab the biscuits and get ourselves settled back in our comfy chair again.

Ready..............

Question: Will I put weigh on during this journey

Answer: Yep 100% you will. (There is probably 1% that doesn't)

Sorry but we need to face the facts. Let me give you some background information regarding my weight through my life up to this point.

So as a teenager and young adult I never worried about my weight, I didn't ever weigh myself and I have no idea how much I weighed, I can't remember what clothes size I was, it just wasn't something that was important to me or my friends we were just getting on living our lives, we didn't have any Social Media so there was no comparison trap to speak of, the worse we probably had (I don't recall any such moments) was Tracey (made up name) at the youth club who was having a bad day. As I say it wasn't on our radar.

In my early 20's is when I had my 3 children, obviously I did put weight on during this time but again I didn't own scales and I honestly don't remember it being a problem. That was up until I had my third child when people started to comment that I had put weight on and maybe I should go do something about it.

Now this was the start to the slippery slope, I did not know this at the time but now I live intuitively I can see this was the start of my relationship with diet culture.

Now lets remember that the people close to me that had wanted me to do something about my weight were doing this from a good place, they were also living in diet culture. So off I went to Weight Watchers, this would have been about 6 months after my son was born, at the time I weighed just over 13 stone and was a size 14. Looking back that really doesn't seem that bad. Anyway after 3 month I had got myself down to about 10 stone was back in a size 10/12 and everyone was happy (including me). Now sadly, I did get divorced and through the stress of that I lost a lot of weight unintentionally, I won't bore you with all the gory details, so my weight went down to under 9 stone and I was wearing size 8/10 clothes, I stayed at this weight for a good 5 years and then slowly I put weight on. Again looking back now that was a good thing, I was actually too thin and not at all healthy.

Please remember thin does not always equal healthy or happy.

Being happy, having a stable income and living my life, going on holidays and eating out of course my weight had crept up a bit so off I went to Slimming World, after having a little dalliance with Slim Fast (I do not recommend that at all) it worked and I lost the weight I wanted to but then my work became more sedentary and on the weight went again, back to Slimming World, you get the picture.

Let's move now to the present day, I have over the last two years put quite a lot of weight on, which in the beginning really did get me down, to be honest I still have days where it gets me down. However, I am the fittest and the healthiest I have ever been I have never done as much regular exercise as I do now, we have the dogs so they get walked and I swim in our pool We live in a country that it absolutely bursting with fresh produce that you just can't help but eat well, there really isn't a take away option so everything we eat I make from scratch.

So you are losing weight I hear you ask, well the answer to that is nope!

It doesn't matter what I do I lose a few pounds and then I end up exactly where I started. So I started to explore Intuitive Eating and Living and do you know it made so much sense. So I have ditched diet culture and all its restrictions, we can see looking back across my history that I am not a naturally fat person but I have come to the conclusion that at the moment this is how my body needs to be to help me through this journey.

I see other women around me who all of a sudden seem to be losing weight but they are all on the other side of their Menopause journey and when they were smack in the middle of their journey they also carried extra weight.

There is definitely a pattern, so I have stopped stressing about it, I continue to exercise because it is good for my mental health, it makes me feel good and I know that it is keeping my body healthy and strong going through this journey. It will also have a positive affect on my bone health which is important as I get older. I continue to read as much as I can about nutrition, I listen to Podcasts of Registered Nutritionalists, I try to live Intuitively this includes exercise as well as food. In the last year my weight has stayed exactly the same so again I firmly believe that this is where it needs to be for now.

I am confident that as I come out the other side that my weight will then go back to its normal set point of where it wants to be that's best for me.

Weight is always going to be a difficult subject as it is something that we talk about constantly, sometimes we are not even aware but diet culture is around us everywhere and it is very clever, as there is a lot of money to make in this industry so you see it all the time and you don't realise. I have read numerous books about

Intuitive eating over the last year and I feel I have a good understanding of it and could talk about it confidently but I still sometimes get caught out by the clever diet culture marketing.

Also, its about reprogramming your brain. If you think back to being a child how much time did you spend thinking about food, weight and clothes size?

I am guessing the answer to that question is you didn't give it any thought, as a child your meals are planned and made by a parent/carer there is no thought process for you, if you are hungry you eat. Babies are fabulous at this, they know exactly when they have had enough and will blow bubbles in their milk, equally if there bodies need fuel, because thats what it is, they will most defiantly let you know they are hungry.

So can we use this information as adults, YES is the answer. Its not easy as you have to unlearn all the diet culture that has been programmed into your head. I know you are thinking I haven't been programmed into anything, Mmmm well lets have a look at these statements.

> No carbs before Marbs
>
> I have a wedding coming up I am being 'good'
>
> I want to wear my bikini on holiday I am going to cut out bread
>
> I need to lose a few pounds so I am going to fast for the next few weeks
>
> Susan in the office has just started WW and is looking great I think I will try (sorry again Susan!)

I am sure there are lots more if we think about it but you get the idea, this is language that is used around us all the time and so our brains naturally go here without even thinking.

Now I think that you have to be careful, this is all well and good if FOR YOU it is the right time to have a look and research Intuitive Eating. It's not for everyone and you may still want to lose weight and that is absolutely fine. There is no judgement here, the anti diet movement has grown over the last year but like everything it has become very loud and inclusive but do you know what just as you have the right to be a person of any size and be happy, if you are not happy you also have the right to lose weight healthily. I find myself getting quite cross when I read things about how people shouldn't lose weight because honestly we are completely individual and we have to make that decision for our selves and it is dependant on so many variables.

For me, because this book is my journey that I wanted to share, I wanted to understand my body because quite frankly somedays it feels like it is falling apart and so my learning journey has lead me to this point in time. Now I would love to be a little thinner, I am sure my knees would appreciate it and it would be lovely to pop into a shop and grab that pretty top knowing it will fit, these outings do get me down, but I also appreciate that at the moment my body is going through a huge change and although it is designed to do this, just the same as it is for breathing, maybe it just needs to be this weight right now.

As I said before I have maintained this weight no matter what I have done but I haven't got any bigger either. So I will continue to eat healthy, workout because it makes me feel good and I am confident that when my body needs to let go of some of this weight it will do so.

I will not stress about it as that will only make everything worse.

CHAPTER 11

SLEEP

Yawn.

Interesting, as I sit down to write this chapter about sleep, I have had two nights of not much sleep.

How can you be this tired and not sleep I frequently ask myself. It's quite normal these days for me to be yawning my head off at seven o'clock in the evening but by the time I go to bed at ten, I can rarely make it much past this time, I am awake.

I have a little ritual that I like to do when I go to bed to help induce sleep, I found a that listening to books rather than reading them helps me drift off, also I discovered a great yoga breath technique that 90% of the time really helps.

I always make sure that my phone is in Do Not Disturb mode from 10pm so that I am not distracted by the world. I do always have my phone near me, I think the fact that I live in a different country from the rest of my family means that I feel better if it close. It will ring if anyone on my favourite list rings me in an emergency. Peace of mind is a great sleep inducer!

Sleeping position? Why is she going to talk about how to sleep I can hear you saying but honestly I am as mystified as you are. Remember how you used to sleep as a child or teenager or to be honest any age before this exciting Menopausal Journey began. Well exactly, you don't and can't because quite frankly you just went to bed and slept.

But now, all of a sudden that doesn't happen, some nights I can get into bed, snuggle down and sleep no problem, haha I am making myself laugh now, this is not very often! Other nights I get into bed and then I am thinking, where does this arm or hand usually go, it feels very awkward, like its someone else, why is my knee hurting in this position, it didn't last night and so it goes on. When did this change happen, I have no idea but all of a sudden snuggling down can be extremely problematic.

Also of course there is the feet thing!

Yes you know they have to be out of the cover, if it hot, if its minus 4 whatever the temperature the feet have to be out. Sometimes you doubt yourself and bring them back in to the warmth of the duvet only for them to have to go out again a few moments later, I was going to say minutes but I don't think they last that long.

Now I have written that and read it back I hope there are some of you out there reading this saying YES! thats exactly it, otherwise it will just be the rantings of a mad woman.

So the yoga breathing, I know I have already talked about this is a previous chapter but it really is very good so I am giving myself permission to repeat the information.

Yoga Breathing Technique to help with sleep

- Firstly get yourself in a comfortable position
- Next just take some deep breathes and have the intention to sleep (by this I mean think that this will work and that you will go to sleep)
- Now take a breath in slowly while counting to 5. Remember slowly,

    1............2............3..........4..........5

- Hold that breath for the count of 5. Again count to 5 slowly this is all about taking time,

    1...........2............3...........4..........5

- Now Slowly (you are getting the idea I am sure) breath out while counting down from 5

    5..........4..........3............2..........1

- Repeat this 5 time.

You should now drift off to sleep. Don't give up on the first try if it doesn't quite work as you hope, these things take time especially if you are not used to doing anything like this.

(You could reduce the number down to 3 for example when you first start this if you find counting to 5 a bit much, I don't want any of you turning blue and running out of breath, thats not going to be conducive for a restful nights sleep.)

So once you are asleep, brilliant, you will be for the whole night and wake up in the morning ready to face the day...................Err no, this is not a Disney movie.

For me I will probably be asleep for maybe an hour, then I wake up to roll over, why? I have absolutely no idea what so ever! But of course now I am awake, I have to go through the process again of trying to work out where this arm should go, why can't I feel my hand (yep thats another symptom , I will talk about that a little more in the Chapter about Aches and Pains, I bet you can't wait!).

So now I am comfortable I can drop back off to sleep? Nope, because now I need to go to the loo. I mean how annoying is that, after all the reorganising, so I shall ignore it, after all I haven't drunk anything I have been asleep.

Pah! Good luck with that, off I go to the loo.

So then it starts again with the snuggling down. Can you see how this is going and of course I don't roll over once in the night oh no, some nights I basically feel that I am rolling over continuously, its no wonder that I wake up completely exhausted.

Other things that keep me awake are;

The moon, sometimes it is just so bright

The dogs, they might hear a sound that sets them off

The dogs, they cuddle up and are just too hot

My Husband, the snoring

My Husband, the not snoring- this can be just as worrying why is he so quiet can I hear him breathing

The dogs, they have laid on my legs and now I can't feel them, have I lost my legs?

The Children, are they all okay have I spoken to the enough, have I spoken to them too much?

Parents, again when did I last speak to them , too soon for another call, maybe its been to long?

Have I got any money in my purse, I cant remember

What day is it tomorrow?

What was the name of the actor we were talking about earlier?

What is that thing I need to remember tomorrow, why didn't I write it down?

You can see my problem, once my brain is going it could literally be thinking about anything at all.

The downside to all this night time excitement is of course that when it is morning and you should be awake, your body can easily get comfortable and you could sleep for England!

So what are the bonuses for no sleeping, as I like to find the positive in as much as I can. Well I have seen some stunning sun rises that are just magical and also because its hot here I can get stuff done while its still relatively cool.

There is always a positive if you look for it.

CHAPTER 12

MOODY

Yep, I think that the analogy of a teenager in reverse works really well for the Menopausal Journey.

I mean, my (our) hormones are just all over the place so to say that on occasion I could be moody just really doesn't cut it. Its not moody like I am sulking it that I am experiencing different moods.

It really is easier I think to say what emotion am I experiencing today, well maybe that should read at the moment because I am a whirl of emotion and they can change very quickly, sometimes so quickly I don't even notice, it is subtle .

Maybe the title for this chapter should read emotional rather than moody because the word moody makes me think grumpy and that isn't really something I feel very often.

In fact lets look up the word and see what it says;

Moody *adjective*

> *teenagers tend to get a bad name for being moody and irresponsible; unpredictable, temperamental, emotional, volatile, capricious, changeable, mercurial, unstable, fickle, flighty*

Nope, I was right first time, Moody is pretty spot on I shall stick with it. So lets explore my moods.

Emotions are a very peculiar thing and can change, well for me anyway, due to the smallest thing. I might hear a song on the radio or I could be chatting to someone who says a word or a phrase which resonates with me and then I am off.

Mostly I would say that I am a happy, upbeat, enthusiastic, excitable person. I love to laugh and humour is an important part of my life. It is good to look for the positives even when life gets tricky and believe me, my life has had plenty of ups and downs along the way, thats probably a whole other book!

These 'Moods' however linked to the menopausal journey are completely different and I know through all the research that I have done that many women are put on anti depressants by their doctors but actually they are not depressed they are Menopausal.

I have thought long and hard about whether or not to include these next few sentences as I am not an expert as we have already accepted but I do want to keep being completely honest and transparent with you. After all that's exactly what the book is all about so, I want to highlight that if you do decide to go to see your GP and they do wish to put you on antidepressants I would like to suggest that you step back and maybe get a second opinion before you start taking pills. Don't get me wrong they can really make a difference if you are depressed but through researching this subject I have come across many women who's doctors Googled Menopause in front of them in the surgery as they don't have any specialist training in this particular field. I hope that there are lots of GP's that can tell me that is wrong but only a few days ago I read about a lady who had this exact problem and she wasn't depressed at all. It gives food for thought I think.

Anyway, back to me.......

This is what is can be like, this by the way is an example of it at its worse;

Morning has arrived, might have been a good sleep night, I don't think this has any impact on my mood, I have tried to see if there is a pattern but so far no.

As I open my eyes I know that the cloud has descended, this is exactly how it feels, like during the night at some point a big fat sad cloud has come along attached itself to the top of my head and there it has decided to stay for awhile. The length of time is never the same so these days I just go with it. As I said before I am a great one for saying things out loud to my hubby , so I will announce to him, today I am sad. We have been doing this for some time now so he knows what I mean and probably knows what's coming just as much as I do.

So I am sad, but it's not like when something sad happens and you feel the sad emotion for that event, oh no, I am sad about absolutely everything, and I am really really sad. Everything I think about makes me feel a little bit worse, usually if its a really bad bout we go and do something, go out for the day, into the outdoors, go to the cinema anything really that can act as a distraction. Feeling sad is extremely draining.

As I am sad and then drained by the sad I become tearful, this is when I miss my children and family the most. I will cry over anything good, bad and in the middle it really doesn't have to have any significance to anything. Literally the wind could be blowing in a different direction and that will be enough to set me off. (I have to add here that I have always been a cryer, for both happy and sad situations)

On days like this I try to keep myself isolated from all people apart from my hubby, I really have no idea if this is the correct way to deal with it but it works for me, there is nothing worse than being with people and then wanting to cry because they offered you a glass of water!

Exercise really helps with this, now I am not sure whether it is because it distracts my brain or whether its those happy endorphins, probably a combination of both but a good Yoga session along with a dog walk really does make me feel better, I still feel sad, but I can cope with it.

Usually, for me, this sad lasts a few days. The first day will be the worst and then the next couple I can feel the cloud beginning to lift and then I will catch myself laughing or singing, its amazing how the singing stops as soon as the sad hits, all I want is complete silence. So yes the singing is back as is the laughter and then I know that I am feeling better again.

As I said at the beginning of this explanation, this is the worst it can be. Sometimes it can be just for a few hours, I thought it was best to give you the worse case scenario that I have experienced, I am guessing that sadly there are a few of you out there that have experienced worse and my heart goes out to you.

As horrible as this is for me to get through, it is difficult for my husband too, another reason why I think our menfolk should read up on all things Menopausal, I mean he doesn't know exactly how I feel, it's hard to explain completely but he is the one who has to navigate it, is it the right time to ask if I want a cup of tea, should he tell me my hair looks nice, you get the idea.

He really does have a lot of patience, thank goodness. I have to say my sons are also very good with me, sometimes I will send them random I love you messages. They always reply with some flippant answer, which makes me laugh and is exactly what I need.

I have read lots of information regarding hormones and how this sad mood is linked and there are of course different drugs you can get prescribe to help with this but I am not one for taking tablets. I don't like taking a painkiller for a headache let alone anything else, I have always been extremely wary and aware that what ever you are putting in your body that is manmade even if it for good will always have some sort of side affect so I avoid prescribe drugs as much as I can.

So if I am not taking anything for the moods is there something else I could do, well apparently Chickpeas are one of the amazing foods along with a few others that can give our bodies oestrogen and this is the hormone that we are losing as we go through this journey. So chickpeas it is then, well I can tell you we have eaten chickpeas in many forms and although I love them I am sick to death of them.

Please no more, and to be perfectly honest they didn't have any impact on the sad mood.

So what I decided on as a plan of action was to do nothing, let the mood come over me and work through it, I know it won,t be around for long, I know that this is just another part of the process that my body is going through and as long as it doesn't become any worse and as long as my husband can still live with me with this symptom then go with the flow is how it will be.

Strangely the other kind of mood that I seem to have to cope with quite often is of a no mood. When I don't really feel anything, now at one point in my life I did have a kind of break down and during this time I experience the no mood but that was more of a don't care no mood, basically my brain/body shut down as it couldn't take anymore is the easiest way to describe it. This no mood is different to that though it is more like....... indifference I suppose. It's like I am watching and listening to what is going on around me but I don't want to be involved or take part in it. It is quite a strange one and thankfully I don't have this very often but thought it was worth mentioning just incase you are feeling like this.

Weird moods and a Menopausal Journey seem to just go hand in hand.

What can we do? As I said earlier for me the answer is nothing, I just like to notice the feeling, acknowledge it if you like and wait for it to pass. Then when it happens again I am like, ah okay here you come I know this feeling and I have the knowledge to know there is nothing wrong, this is part of my journey and it will pass.

CHAPTER 13

OUCH!

So along with everything that I have shared already there is I am afraid more.

I know, I am sorry, I want this book to be uplifting, positive, helpful, dare I say life changing and liberating and so far I have shared a lot of problems, but hopefully between all the symptoms that I have shared you are beginning to see that it normal, every woman will do this.

It is completely normal and just part of being a woman.

We need to find our smiles to get through it but also for our own sanity.

Lets put the mug that had our cup of tea and the plate that had our slice of cake on it into the sink and lets grab the chocolates and a glass of your favourite tipple (doesn't have to be alcoholic), get comfy again in your favourite spot and tackle this next chapter. I have called it ouch! because it is about all the wonderful aches and pains that I have developed.

Today as I sit here writing these are my aches and pains. I would like to add that today for me is an absolute magnificent sort of a day. Mood normal, energy levels normal.

- Ache in right shoulder
- Stiff right knee
- Weak left ankle
- Sore hips
- Strange sort of ovary ache

‣ Aching lower back

What a lovely collection of aches and pains you are thinking I am sure. I actually think I have forgotten a couple, its not a brain fog day, maybe if I get up and walk around a bit I will find the others!

Ah yes there we go I remembered another one, it only happens at night thats why I couldn't feel it as I was writing.

‣ Carpal Tunnel in both my wrists.

Ah the joys!

So before you start feeling sorry for me its fine, mostly they don't all hurt all at the same time, they don't even hurt all the time and I have ways of dealing with it, so its not like my life is being directly affected by any of these it just that they are there.

I remember once when I was really young and worked in an Old Peoples Home (Care Home's they are called now) an old man told me that he liked waking up with aches and pains because that's how he knew he was alive! I don't think I am anywhere near that close to death but I do understand more what he meant now, I think when he told me I was so young, (teenager) so busy getting on with my life that I was a bit blasé about what he had said.

‣ theres another, clicking knees! (I have always had clicking knees but they are worse now)

Anyway, lets explore each one firstly the shoulder ache. I really have no idea why this started to happen, just one morning I woke up with what I would have described as a stiff shoulder, you know, you have laid in a strange position while you were asleep and it feels tight when you wake. It started like that, although we have already established that I don't sleep very well, so a deep awkward sleep is not really possible. So there it was a stiff shoulder, that stayed and stayed and well it's still there although now I would say it is more of a constant ache rather than stiff. I do Yoga regularly and I do find that it can ease the ache but it never really goes away completely and then the next day its back.

The Stiff right knee, well this one is a fun one. I have over the last year been exercising more and more, finding what I like and exploring how my body responds, nothing rushed and no pressure to achieve anything except healthy movement. I have discovered that I really enjoy resistant workouts, I have my kettle bell and Dumbbells and it has really amazed me how with regular practice your body can get stronger and actually is much more capable than you think. It is always your brain that gives up first not your body. So I found a new workout plan, I like to change them around so that I don't get bored, it was a 28 day one, all the moves were ones that I already knew, nothing different apart from how the 28 days were set out and the combinations. Up until now I tended to do a full body workout but this plan meant you had an arm and abs day, a leg day and then a full body day. All was going well , I was enjoying it, I had to modify some of the moves but thats completely normal and I didn't always complete all the reps and again I was fine with this it was something new and I didn't want to go mad and then had to have extra rest days due to injury. Week two went passed, all good then half way through week 3, my right knee began to hurt every time I did anything like a squat or lunge. So I stopped, had a few rest days , then tried again. Nope it wasn't going to play, so I stopped the 28 day plan and thought thats fine I will just do Yoga and swimming both can be low impact on knees. Here we are, 3 months on and my right knee is still hurting. I am still swimming and doing Yoga as if I do nothing it gets stiff and then thats worse but it doesn't seem to be improving so thats another one that I have collected.

Weak left ankle, no big story with this one, got up one morning went downstairs in the normal fashion, nothing fancy and thought Mmmm that feels strange and strange it has been ever since, it doesn't hurt, its just every now and then usually if I am going up and down steps it cracks and feels like it might give way, it hasn't done yet thank goodness, that could be embarrassing!

Sore hips, probably better described as an ache rather than sore. I know I have hips. I am not old, I am 48 but you do get to an age, I don't actually know when it is because it just arrives and you are doing it but you can't remember when it started, when overtime you sit down or stand up and a strange sort of sigh/groan escapes from your mouth. You try not too but it's out before you can stop it, well I think the hip thing is just like that really. Just another body part wearing out! Oh deep joy.

I think I should have taken my own advise and got a glass of wine when I suggested getting yours, maybe not, you would have been reading complete gibberish by now!

Ovary Ache, this one used to worry me a bit, I have had it a long time, maybe five years ish, nope thats nonsense its more like ten years. I know that there is absolutely nothing wrong with me and that it is just a symptom on the list but it used to worry me. Its a strange place for an ache and yes we all have them when we are having our period but to have them at random times is not the best. Again, I have been check by a doctor and I know I am fine and I have read up about it and yes lots of people suffer with it and it is just that a menopausal symptom. For me remedied by painkillers when its really bad.

Lower back ache, this is the same as the hips, just I am not a teen-ager anymore and if I do something really strenuous then the next few days I feel it. Its the quiet sigh/groan again.

And the last item on my list, Carpel Tunnel in both wrists, now this is a joy!

I have had this five or six years, when it is cold it is much worse so living in a warm/hot country is very helpful. When it first started I moaned about it a lot, it is tedious and annoying, I wake in the morning and both my hands have pins and needles where they are asleep but it is really painful, sometimes it wakes me up in the night. I bought wrist supports and went to the doctors, my doctor gave me physio moves that you can do to help and told me that the wrist supports would help but only wear them at night. Great I thought, did the physio moves, wore the support, it has helped a little. I don't wear the supports these days very often but I do still wake up with numb painful hands and the only thing that helps the pain and helps fast is a basic technique that a good friend of mine told me about. What you do is roll to the edge of the bed, through your arms over so that all the blood can rush to your fingers and then wiggle said fingers fast. I mean is does look at little strange and it does make the dogs jump sometimes but as we have already established my hubby is a saint and is quite used to me doing strange things.

Our house is a fun place to be!

CHAPTER 14

FUN

Well, I feel like we have been very serious and tackled a lot of subjects that are a bit full on and remember this is not a disease this is just the natural part of being a woman so I think we need to do something fun for a bit.

What shall we do?

As much as I would like you to keep on reading my book, I mean thats the reason I wrote it, I think we all need a time out. So lets have some Me Time.

Go back to the Me Time chapter and find one or maybe a few things that you really want to do right now and then let's do them.

Make sure that you smile all the time, might get tricky if you re going to do face mask, but smile anyway crack that mask, enjoy it and then lets meet back here tomorrow and we can carry on discussing the other exciting things we have to look forward to to like irregular periods and other peoples opinions!

For me, I am going to make a big cup of peppermint tea, have a bath with a face mask.

Enjoy your Me Time and see you tomorrow X

CHAPTER 15

PERIODS

This is a very no hoes barred chapter, so if you are slightly squeamish in any way just bear this in mind as I wanted to be brutally honest. I mean there is no point in sharing my journey to help you feel normal if I cut corners or make it sparkly and pretty if its not.

So here goes.......

Periods or Star Week, Time of the Month, Women's stuff, whatever you feel comfortable with, I mean we can't talk Menopause Journey and not discuss this. After all this is one of the most crucial pieces of the puzzle.

So this is my personal journey remember so I can only go by how my body is working or not depending in how you look at it, I think mine is dull. Don't get me wrong, dull is good, I have heard some complete horror stories of what women have had to go through so I am happy to stick with dull.

So what am I up to, well nothing much really. My periods last three days generally, this has been the case for the last ten years I would say, day one is spotting, day two is a full on bleed but not particularly heavy, day three spotting and then jobs done!

I know right, easy peasy, well that is most of the time.

The one change I did have to make was to stop using Tampons and go back to sanitary towels, now I will use Tampons on the odd occasion like if I am swimming but actually these days I tend just not to swim. I found that I became very uncomfortable using Tampons and I also found that on my full flow day I leaked quite a lot and no one wants that do they.

So Sanitary towels it is and then life is much more relaxed, if I have to miss one day of swimming every month during the summer, well that's fine I can live with that, no drama.

Then about four years ago, it might be longer, I can't really remember now, my periods started to become unpredictable, up until this point I was very regular, now sometimes it can be every six weeks or maybe I will miss a month and then we are off again, just as I think a pattern is forming it goes again. Now I must say once again that I am lucky in as far as mine are either monthly or more spread out, I am very aware that lot's of women have them really close together or just bleed continuously so I can't grumble. So now for me it can almost be like an unwanted surprise!

I just make sure that I always have a supply of sanitary towels with me and then I am good to go.

Well, up until just this week that was the case, then all change! We were on holiday, we only had three days left before we were due to fly home. I woke up and knew immediately that my period was imminent, we just know right. So I thought to myself that fine, it will only be the last three days no drama, I have everything I need, it would have been better it could have waited until I returned home but there it is.

Oh No! I could not have been more wrong, this period came with vengeance I have not experienced since I was a teenager, minus the pain, thank goodness. This was full on bleed from the get go. Okay I am thinking to myself I can do this even if the three days are like this its not a problem and then I am home. Nope, it was a huge problem, it was a full on bleed for three day and then it continued, it actually continued for five days full, the heaviest period I can remember and then it stopped as quickly as it started.

Well, thats not so bad I can hear you thinking, but actually it was horrendous, the sheets in every place we stayed for the last three days were white, yes WHITE! Crisp and fresh like a blinking Persil advert!

Then of course to get home we had a ten and a half our flight, again thats no problem I can hear you saying, but it was, yes I could sleep and rest, yes I was sitting down but oh my god! The bleed got even heavier, I don't know if it has something to do with the air pressure or flying or whether this was just how it would have been but I can tell you I have never been happier to get off a plane!

The worse thing was that even though I was over prepared and visited the toilet regularly throughout the flight I leaked on to my clothes, I was mortified and tearful, well the hormones, you can image!

Actually, as a side note, we were watching Grey's Anatomy last night, do you watch it? Anyway Bailey was feeling out of sorts, very hot and tearful and so she had her bloods done, the results, she was peri menopausal, all she said as she sat down was, " **Oh all the emotions**" My Hubby looked at me and smiled and said that he was going to call me Bailey from now on, in that small sentence she completely summed up how it feels to be on this journey.

All the emotions.

Anyway back to me getting off this flight, now I have to wrap my cardigan around my waist as I am completely paranoid that everyone knows my predicament. My hubby offers me his hoody too as its cold but better to be cold than for people to know. As always my husband is completely calm, tells me its fine, no one can see, I am sure it has happened to other people, don't worry.

DON'T WORRY! Does he know me? I worry about everything all the time, even if it hasn't happened or might not happen or is happening someone else and then I cry because of cause that always helps! I say again **ALL the emotions**.

So I get home in one piece, the world hasn't stopped turning and all is well but this period did as I said before carry on in this manner for another two days at which point when it had finished I was absolutely exhausted. Everyone was expecting us to return from our holiday rested and I look like I need a holiday.

So now I have questions?

Is this how my periods are going to be moving forward?

Was this like a last hurrah and now its finished? (Fingers crossed on this one)

Did it just get affected by the flight? (I shall be researching this and reporting back)

Or was it just another weird one off and then I shall go back to carrying on in my normal fashion?

I have absolutely no idea, but like everything with the journey I will try and step back and observe as I know I have no control and this is something that my body needs to do.

Right then, I have researched the whole, does flying make my flow heavier and I was surprised to find out that actually the consensus is no. If anything your flow will be lighter. So thats just blown that theory out of the water. All the information that I could find and I read a lot, stated that traveling and long haul flights can mess up your normal menstrual cycle, causing you to be early or late, this is down to the stress placed on your body, not that you are stressed but apparently different time zones and just the act of travelling is enough to put your body in stress and so it reacts by affecting your cycle. Absolutely nowhere does it say that the flow will get heavier so that means I am left with these questions;

Is this how my periods are going to be moving forward?

Was this like a last hurrah and now its finished? (Fingers crossed on this one again)

Or was it just another weird one off and then I shall go back to carrying on in my normal fashion?

I guess I will just have to wait and see what happens next. Over the next month I am flying two more time, although they are not long haul flights, so I will be able to observe if this has any affect, I guess once I get back into my normal life rhythm at home I will be able to see if this heavy flow is here to stay.

I have to say I am really hoping that it was my last hurrah and they will stop. I have just worked out that I have been having periods for thirty three years! WOW! I think thats enough now, don't you?

(I just said that our loud to myself, haha, I am quite old, thats not something I think about often, age is just a number and I don't think it should constrain you to stop or start anything but when you say it our loud sometimes it catches you- I must be having a good day today as there was no cue tears! Bonus!!)

So to update this chapter and keep it real, the periods have changes again, they really are all over the place, because the last one was so horrendous and I don't want to be caught out ever I thought I would start tracking my periods on my phone, yes if you weren't aware this is a thing, I have an iPhone but I would image that Androids have the same facility. Anyway you log in when you have your period any symptoms you experience and then it can give you an idea of when they next one will rear is ugly head!

So I am two months in from starting the logging and so far it has been spot on (no pun intended!) but now I have found that for the week leading up to my period and the week after I am spotting, no big deal you think, but actually yes its a major big deal, Why? well I will tell you.

Not only am I spotting but I am suffering from spots, like a teen-ager, cramping, breast tenderness, mood swings and of course the spotting is heavy enough that I need a sanitary towel, so now I feel like my period is lasting 3 weeks, joy!

The worst bit with all of this is that I am tired, we discussed the tired before and its awful so now I have three weeks of tired, which in turn makes me light headed, nauseous and weak. Are you getting the picture now?

So what can I do, I honestly at the time of writing this do not know, I still am firmly in the no medication camp, I will get through it, I am listening even more to my body, resting if I need to, going to bed ridiculously early if need be, laying in longer than I normally would, being vocal so my husband knows why I am the way I am. I have stopped all exercise apart from Yoga as this helps still my anxiety and palpitations and generally makes me feel like I can cope with the world.

Lastly, I am making myself get on with living and telling myself, I am not ill I am peri menopausal and it will pass. It does help, but if I am honest it is a struggle.

CHAPTER 16

WHAT ARE YOU EATING?

"Food Glorious Food"

I will stop, singing is not my forte but food is an interesting subject. I remember right at the beginning, when I started to read up about Menopause the subject of food came up a lot. There are whole books out there with Menopause diets. All the foods that will replace your oestrogen (you remember the chickpeas!) but I have to say that the food in these books, well some of them, were.............. I think weird really is the best way for me to describe them.

Now, my dad has always said that I am a hippie and to be honest I am really interested and aware of my environment and if I can make something myself, soap for example or recycle something then I am happy to do that. But some of the books I read even made sit back and think wow, if I start eating like this people are going to think I have lost the plot. Now don't get me wrong, I am not driven to please other people, well not these days anyway, but honestly some of the things I read were laughable. I mean whatever we do to keep us on the straight and narrow through this journey has to be sustainable, we have to be able to continue to live as part of the community. I think if I had started to go out for dinner accompanied by tupperware containers of seeds and nutty goodness people would have had their concerns and rightly so.

As with everything, not just Menopause, you have to do whats right and what works for you. I fully encourage everyone to read and learn as much as you can and try things, but also I would encourage you to remember that there never is just one way, so you have to try because what works for me may not work for you.

You know this.

So let's address Superfoods, these are supposed to be individual food items that have amazing benefits if we consume them and I am sure that you have all read about a least one in the last ten years. Some of the claims are quite amazing but actually if you listen or read articles from Registered Nutritionist or Registered Dieticians then the information is completely different, in as far as the super part. Yes the food that have all these magical claims are good for you if eaten as a whole food, not processed, and if eaten as part of a healthy balanced diet. Just because you eat your body weight of Chia Seeds you are not miraculously going to be better.

We have already established right at the beginning of this book that it is not a disease but a process that our bodies need to go through and are designed to go through, our bodies are amazing remember and we can just let it get on with the process. So we are not going to get better, also what would life be like if you had to consume the above amount of Chia Seeds, it really doesn't bare thinking about!

So what other superfoods are there that are supposed to work miracles, these are the ones I have discovered during my research;

>Maca Powder
>Chia Seeds
>Coconut water
>Sea Salt
>Broccoli Sprouts
>Pomegranates
>Chocolate (Raw Cacao)
>Red Wine

So probably not really any surprises in this list, although I don't think I had read about Broccoli Sprouts before, I like broccoli and I am partial to a sprout but this is not making me think yum. Also, look the famous chickpeas are not on this list as they are not classed as a Super food.

Well guess what, non of these are super, they are just ingredients, there is no such thing as a good food or a bad food. Its all just food, it's what you do with the ingredients that counts. Again, this is completely individual to each person, I for example don't ever really have milk, I don't like it, it makes me feel sick if I drink to much, so there is no point in telling me I have to drink it because its good for me because its not it makes me feel sick!

I have a favourite nutritionist called Rhiannon Lambert, I follow her on Instagram and listen to her podcasts and I would highly recommend you do the same if you are interested in this subject as she always speaks sense and regularly on a Monday does a myth busting post, they are always informed and interesting.

What I have learnt not just from Rhiannon Lambert, there are lots of good qualified people out there, is that really you need to keep it simple. If you eat whole foods, the ones that look like their original form and haven't been highly processed then you will get the nutrients from them that help fuel your body.

Now for example Orange juice, sometimes I love a glass of orange juice but I know that really I would be better off eating an orange, a glass of orange juice isn't going to hurt me but as a whole food I get more fuel than if I have it as a drink. Every now again though is fine, if I drank only orange juice this could be a problem.

I hope I am making sense here, we all have discover these things for ourselves, I mean I have already told you about my chickpea chapter but I had to do that to find out for myself, I still eat chick-peas just not obsessively.

Part of learning about Intuitive Eating has helped me with this, as really its about being aware of what you fuel your body with for you without outside influence, we all know that if we eat cake and biscuits and nothing else we are not going to feel our best, but sometimes we have to do this to prove it to ourselves then we can make an informed choice.

Another example I can give you is bread. Now I know bread is very controversial, some people think it is the devil food and it has had very bad press over the last few years but remember there is no bad food. Its all just food. I tend to only eat bread as toast for my breakfast, I am not saying I never eat it at any other time as that would be a lie, but mainly its a breakfast thing, why is that? Well I find if I eat it later in the day it lays heavy in my stomach and I feel uncomfortable so I choose not to eat it as I choose not to feel uncomfortable.

I would encourage everyone to go out and experiment and step back and notice how the food that you are feeding your body with is making you feel, I think you will be surprised, and what have you got to lose?

I don't think, remember this is just my opinion, that you can have a Menopausal Diet, but I do think that if you can eat well, fresh, whole foods with a full and balanced mix then you will feel better, this isn't because it is some kind of magical cure for menopause symptoms. Its the same for everyone, male and female, young and old, fresh whole foods release all the nutrients and vitamins into your body to fuel it and so this means you will feel better.

It is worth keeping a food diary, not to calorie count but to observe how the foods that you are eating are making you feel.

Are you full? Are you bloated? Are you full of energy? Did you make it to the next meal without feeling starving?

You get the idea, have a go, you might be surprised!

I have given you a four weekly table that you can use to help record your feelings about the foods you are eating, remember this is not about calories its about how the fuel you put in your body makes you feel,

Have some fun with it!

Monday	Breakfast	Lunch	Dinner	Snacks
Tuesday				
Wednesday				
Thursday				
Friday				
Saturday				
Sunday				

Monday	Breakfast	Lunch	Dinner	Snacks
Tuesday				
Wednesday				
Thursday				
Friday				
Saturday				
Sunday				

Monday	Breakfast	Lunch	Dinner	Snacks
Tuesday				

Wednesday				
Thursday				
Friday				
Saturday				
Sunday				

Monday	Breakfast	Lunch	Dinner	Snacks
Tuesday				
Wednesday				
Thursday				
Friday				
Saturday				
Sunday				

This is your book, so make as many notes as you need, you can keep coming back to this when you need to.

Once again remember it's all about the feelings you get from the fuel you are eating.

CHAPTER 17

DON'T FORGET
TO STRETCH!

I would like to revisit exercise, I have touched on it in a few chapters but I think like food it's one of those subjects that deserves it's own chapter.

I am not really sure where exactly to start on this one, so I think I will give you little background and then share my last year of exercise .

So background first, the question has to be what exercise do you do? The answer to this would be a nope I don't do exercise at all but this wouldn't be a completely true statement. I haven't done regular consistent exercise throughout my life, I have dabbled here and there and somethings I like and others not so much. Lets explore this a little more, when I was at school I didn't really enjoy PE as a whole but there were elements I enjoyed, Tennis, Hockey and Javelin. I only took part in these at school, never as extra curriculum or at clubs out of school. I have always had it in my head that I am really not good at sports, that I would always come last, be picked last for a team, that sort of thing so the thought of putting myself out there for scrutiny just isn't for me but actually now I know that this is not actually the case.

I can in fact do anything I want to, I just need to do it consistently and have a little self belief and my body will do the rest, your mind always gives in before your body. Once you know this it opens up a whole world of possibilities.

Anyway, so through my adult life I have done exercise classes, water aerobics, spin classes. Spin Classes, these I did not enjoy, have you seen Bridget Jones when she gets off the bike and her legs give out, well that is exactly how I felt!

But do you know now I think I understand why I didn't really get on with any exercise before and it was because I was doing it for the wrong reasons. Let me explain.

What is the reason to do any exercise, well of course it burns calories, so that means you can have that naughty treat and you will lose weight.

Errr no!

You cannot exercise your way out of a bad diet. I have discovered that you do exercise for how it makes you feel. Well how does it make you feel, hot and sweaty? Well yes of course but also, it makes you feel happy, it lifts your mood. It also makes you feel confident in yourself. It really does.

Last year I found by chance Tally Rye on Instagram and because of her philosophy regarding exercise I have had my eyes opened and have changed my thought process from one of, you exercise to lose weight to you exercise for how it makes you feel. Now consistency is still key to a certain extent, you have to understand that as soon as you stop using your body it relaxes, which is absolutely fine, but then you have to start at the beginning and build it up again. Also, absolutely fine!

Let me give you example to explain myself better. Yoga, I have dabbled here and there over the last few years but then I discover a wonderful lady on YouTube recommended by a good friend of mine you can do Yoga at home, she explains everything really clearly and makes sure that you are going at your own speed, this journey is yours so don't compare yourself with anyone else.

(To be honest that goes for all things in life.)

So yes anyway Yoga, when I started I found that I wasn't quite as flexible as I thought I was but with regular practice it is amazing how quickly your body starts to stretch. Over a two week period

I would say I could see a huge difference, that's no long at all is it to see changes. This got me thinking. Then I discovered Tally.

She set up a Best Me Facebook group to encourage everyone to exercise because it is good for you, she set up videos and plans and challenges over a four week period. I was hooked, this was brilliant, I was learning new things and understanding what it was doing for me, let me tell you it is so much more than burning a few calories.

Now as a peri menopausal woman building up my stamina and strength is really important to protect my bone health, sadly as we know as you go through this menopause journey your bone health changes.

So now I am a proud owner of Dumbbells and a kettle bell, I enjoy, yes you read that correctly, I enjoy exercise. Now my weeks are taken up with Yoga, resistant training, swimming when it is warm and walking. Walking is very important and I love being outside, having the dogs is a great motivator as they need their walks every day so even if I am having a really 'Bad' day I know I have to walk them. When I return from my walk I always feel better, it doesn't solve anything or make anything magically disappear but I feel better in myself.

I was really keen when I started out on this part of my learning and so I would exercise six days out of seven only ever allowing myself that one rest day and even then I would walk the dogs, but now as I learned more and moved through this chapter of my life I have slowed it down a bit, I have learnt that rest days are just as important as the exercise days and then your body performs better if you allow it to have the rest days.

So how does this impact on my Menopause Journey I can hear you asking, that's what the book is supposed to be about. Well I think like everything I have chatted about with you, it is just another thing I have learned about that I can use like a tool to get me through the journey. The Yoga helps me to relax and stretch my body which in turn quietens my mind and helps with my aches and pains.

The walking and the swimming gives me quiet and time to contemplate and thing and helps lift my mood.

The resistance training helps to keep my body strong which as I said earlier I understand is good for my bone health as I get older.

So really I feel like is a win win. Anything that helps me feel better about myself and helps me on a low mood day or an aches and pain day has to be a good thing.

Again as in the last chapter I would encourage everyone to get out there and try something. I am not one for the gym, they make me feel super uncomfortable and although I have tried a few times, running isn't my thing, I always feel like I am dying but there are so many other things that you can be doing. Even if walking everyday is all you can manage at the moment then brilliant, it will only ever have a positive impact.

It is just about listening to your body, finding out what works for you and then doing it. It really is that easy.

If I can go from someone who would laugh if you asked do I exercise to some one who looks forward to exercising and I can actually say hand on heart that I enjoy it, then you definitely can do it too.

(It has just occurred to me that I didn't share with you the wonderful YouTube account that I follow for my Yoga. The YouTube channel is called Yoga with Adrienne. There is something for everyone, she has monthly calendars that you can follow with millions of other people around the world, you can find Beginners Yoga and she also has videos that concentrate on individual moves to give you more understanding if you are new to Yoga.)

CHAPTER 18

INTUITIVE LIVING

Intuitive Living sounds very on trend, very mumbo jumbo but I promise you its not.

Actually it probably should be just called Living.

Why? Because thats all we really are doing, every twist and turn or new bit of information that we learn is just part of living. There really is no wrong or right, you have to do what is right for you with the knowledge that you have at that time. You should never judge anyone for their choices as you have no idea what they are going through and what has brought them to this point.

I think that is so important to remember while you are going through your Menopausal Journey, it is just that, it is yours. I have tried to keep this book as light and airy as I can, it is a very heavy subject and some of us out there are really suffering but its is so important to not compare your self with anyone. Just because this is how my journey is progressing does not mean that's how your will go, the solutions and coping mechanism I have found and use work for me, they may not work for you. I would like you to use this book as a starting place, to know that what you are living through is normal, yes completely normal. Yes it is hard, yes there are days when you just want to crawl under your duvet and not come up but that also is completely normal. As soon as you take the pressure off and relax things do ease a little.

Lets put this in some perspective, you may feel reading this that I have got it sussed and have all the answers but you would be wrong, I have read lots and lots and spent hours researching, thank goodness for Google but I am sure I have only just touched on the tip of the iceberg.

Intuitive Living is much the same as Intuitive eating. Its about understanding you. Its about really stepping back and observing, writing a journal everyday and meditating can I think really help with this process.

Why are you acting in a certain way, how does that make you feel, is that how you want to proceed.

When I get up in the morning, I always these days take the time to be grateful for what I have, I do a short meditation and then I will do my chosen exercise for the day depending on how I am feeling. I also like to read for ten minutes and write my list of what I want to achieve during the day. Then I can get on with my day. This all sounds fabulous, serine and fluffy and sometimes it is. It didn't happen over night I have spent the last couple of years trying different things, finding what works and now I have for the most part come to this routine.

Also remember, I am retired so I have time to do these things in the morning, when I was working and had my children at home there is absolutely no way I would have been able to do all of these, maybe one of them. Although thinking about it, sometimes remembering to brush my hair before I left the house was hard work, I do remember once going to work having only put mascara on one eye, I had obviously got distracted. I only noticed when I got home in the evening, not one person had commented on it all day, goodness knows what they must have thought!

Somedays it is so far from this serine routine you could not believe, I could get out of bed, trip over the dog, spill water everywhere when making our morning drink and my day will probably carry on in that vain, I will be saying to my hubby, Its one of those days!

There is always something to bring you back to reality with a bump, yesterday was perfect example of this. We had a really lovely Sunday, very relaxed and chilled I did complete my morning routine, I completely my list for the day and I spent a good portion of my day reading, lovely then I decided I would do some baking, it had been in my head for a while so off I go to make scones. All good until I tried to put the scales in the fridge!

Yes you read that right, the scales in the fridge. I knew then it was time to stop baking and do something else. Before discovering Intuitive Living I would probably have got cross with myself and my stupid brain and pushed myself to keep going, but I know now that if I had done that I would have ended up getting more frustrated, things would have kept going a little bit more bananas and I would have ended up in tears. Now though I can stand still take stock and think okay thats enough for today, stop now before it gets out of hand and come back to it another day.

Yes I acknowledge that I have the luxury of time that working people don't have, but I honestly believe that I if I had known this information when I was working I would have done things differently. Hindsight is a wonderful commodity isn't it!

So Intuitive Living for me, is just really listening and being aware of me. Going at my pace and doing what is right, what feels right for me. No ones life is perfect and every plan has changes to it but if you have a strong base that you can keep referring back to then I believe that it really helps, it has certainly helped me.

It may sound selfish but it really is about you.

This is your journey, you have to get through each day so you need to do what is right for you as much as possible. The one thing that is the most important part of all of this is

YOU

CHAPTER 19

PRESCRIBED DRUGS (FROM YOUR DOCTOR)

So this is a subject that I don't really know anything about as I haven't wanted to go down this road.

I should probably tell you the reason behind this as we are being so open and honest with each other.

Well quite a few years ago now about 7, my mum was diagnosed with Breast Cancer, now at the time of her diagnosis there was rumblings about whether or not the fact that she had been on HRT for so long could have been a cause, as it was they decided no it wasn't, coincidentally at around the same time there were articles on the news about the same thought process. I do have to point out that none of this was ever confirmed as far as I am aware, so please don't let me put you off, I am NOT saying that HRT causes Breast Cancer.

(Mum is absolutely fine by the way and had her all clear and has been clear with no hiccups ever since.)

But what I am saying is that for me personally, that bit of doubt had planted a seed in my head and it has stayed there, I am also a person who never takes pills of any kind, I think I have told you this already, so as I said I won't take a painkiller I am not likely to take HRT!

I do want to give a rounded view for you all though, so I am going to go away and do some research and then I will come back and tell you what I have found out. Please remember that I am only going to tell you what I have found from reading articles, books and listening to podcasts, I am not going off to become a doctor or a medical expert in this field so you will have to go and see a doctor and professionals if you want to explore this route as part of your journey.

So this is what I found out. Where ever I looked and whatever I read the first option that is presented is always HRT.

HRT for those of you that don't know introduces oestrogen back into your body, this is what we are lacking and why we have all these wonderful symptoms. Now I did say above that in my head there is a personal connection between HRT and Breast Cancer and actually on the NHS website it clearly states that in some cases there is an associated risk with Breast Cancer in some women. So for me that doubt is enough, but you must of course get your own advise from your doctor and make your own decision, we are all different.

The next option that comes up to help us is Vaginal Oestrogen, now I had to research more as I had no idea what this was/is. Well it is in pessary form and helps you if your vagina becomes dry, painful and itchy! Oh good lord, I really don't want to suffer from that one.

Next on the list was low dose antidepressants to help if you have been diagnosed depressed, I did find a couple of alternatives if you are suffering from low mood rather than depression, these were Yoga, Tai Chi and CBT (Cognitive Behavioural Therapy).

Then I found some information about prevention of Osteoporosis, which is the following;

> HRT (!)
> Exercise- 21/2 hrs a week aerobic / 2 days a week minimum strength training
> Healthy Diet- particularly calcium
> Sunlight - Vitamin D
> Stop Smoking
> Reduce Alcohol intake

> Take Calcium and Vitamin D tablets if you think
> you maybe deficient

I did find some mention of herbal alternatives but they were always accompanied by a caveat of there is no findings that they help and they could cause more problems for example Breast Cancer.

So I think and you may agree that this is a bit depressing, basically if we go to the doctors and /or try and find out the answer for ourselves the answer 9 times out of 10 is going to be HRT, that's even the answer for the treatment for Osteoporosis, I mean I kind of feel that we don't really have many options.

For me I am going to stick with what I am doing now, manage my symptoms as best I can.

I was hoping that I would be able to give you all a bit more information and some options but I guess they just aren't there for us yet. Hopefully there is someone out their in a lab trying to find the answer for us. Fingers crossed.

Please please please though, do lots of research yourselves and so seek medical advise always.

CHAPTER 20

GENERAL DAY TO DAY

At the moment day to day is difficult, I just wanted to share how a normal day would run for me, this book so far has split everything into separate segments but of course when you are living it everything can happen at once.

Yesterday was for me a perfect day to share with you as I had so much going on peri menopause wise as well as spending New Years day with my husband, we were out for the day spending time together, exploring which is something we both enjoy so all good you may think, well the exploring and spending time was but everything else that was going on, not so much.

The day started as normal, woke up feeling exhausted, wrists hurting, pins and needles in my hands, stiff right knee, left ankle and left shoulder. I always try to start the day in a positive way so thought about what I was grateful for, did a little journalling and some yoga.

All the time time rumbling in the background, my heart palpitating softly, not intense just there in the background, my left arm is uncomfortable, it doesn't hurt, my brain is whirring, is there something wrong, am I going to be ill do I need to go to the hospital. No I am fine, remember women have strokes more than heart attacks, most happen at night and this is morning, this is just a panic attack, peri menopause symptoms, breath.

Recently I read that we have something like 10,000 thoughts a day!?! I think when I feel like this I must be having 10,000 thoughts a minute.

During the drive out, the exploring, the laughter the stopping for lunch no matter what we have done today in the back of my head running like a voice monologue is this.

my heart palpitating softly, not intense just there in the background, my left arm is uncomfortable, it doesn't hurt, my brain is whirring, is there something wrong, am I going to be ill do I need to go to the hospital. No I am fine, remember women have strokes more than heart attacks, most happen at night and this is morning, this is just a panic attack, peri menopause symptoms, breath.

Just over and over again, never stopping. To be honest it is absolutely exhausting. I can't keep telling my husband every time I feel this otherwise we literally would not discuss anything else and also I don't want to be focussing on this, it is so negative, I want to distract myself so that I forget. Remember of course that your brain gets bored at about 45 minutes and just has to think of something else, so I know that I will have some respite from the constant drone of worry. It takes a lot of effort to enjoy a day and have fun when it just there in your head.

I can of course add to my brain reminder that we did this yesterday and the day before and for as long as I can remember and I haven't fallen off the planet yet.

And why is that, because there is nothing wrong with me, no illness, no disease, nothing.

Its just "Menopause"! Just.....................

For all of us living this everyday I am sending you the biggest well done. For getting up and keeping going. It would be easy to stay in bed and let it come over you in a wave but is that going to help, does it make it go away? Well for me no, it would still be there when I got up so instead I start everyday with a positive mindset and tackle it head on, it will not take my days from me, after all we won't get them back and there are people out there who are ill or do have diseases and they don't have tomorrow.

I do always let my husband know if it really is a particularly bad one, if there is a difference or an extra to the constant monologue above. So like today I had all of this going on in my head while we enjoyed what actually was one of the best day we have had for a while, but also today I was sad, with my cloud descending, as the morning went by the sad got worse and got a hold. Which meant that as we were driving in the car on route for our fun day of exploring the tears arrived, not crying or sobbing, after all I have nothing to be sad about, but just tears falling from my eyes down my face, like a waterfall. This lasted probably half an hour so I had to tell him, it was a bad day.

I can honestly say that although this sounds horrendous as you read it, I know I am not suffering as bad as some and also I don't want you to feel sorry for me, it is more about understanding me.

I can't go round explaining all of the above, well the whole book intact to everyone I meet so I guess sometimes I might come over as unsociable or boring or strange but I am doing all this

my heart palpitating softly, not intense just there in the background, my left arm is uncomfortable, it doesn't hurt, my brain is whirring, is there something wrong, am I going to be ill do I need to go to the hospital. No I am fine, remember women have strokes more than heart attacks, most happen at night and this is morning, this is just a panic attack, peri menopause symptoms, breath.

while I am chatting to you, asking you how you are. Listening and be supportive if you are having a bad time, laughing if you are telling me something funny. As I said above it is exhausting and I am looking forward to it stopping, or easing a bit. It would be lovely to just have one day where my brain thinks of something else all day long.

I can but dream…………..

CHAPTER 21

CONCLUSION

So I wanted to write a conclusion at the end of my book but the thing is of course that I am nowhere near the end of my journey so how can I write a conclusion?

I have thought about this for days, actually I think it has been more like a month. As you know I haven't written a book before so this is all new territory for me and I just wanted to help people, women, by telling my story so I just sat down an started typing but the more I wrote the more I started to understand more about what I am going through, I actually understand myself better and am much more aware of what I am doing and feeling on a daily basis.

Over the last year I have read many self help books and listened to podcasts to try and understand this more and it appears that actually if I had just started to write a diary or journalling regularly then I probably would have ended up in exactly the same place.

I guess we will never really know, I am also rather proud that I have sat and shared this experience with you all, I really do hope someone is reading this! It has given me more confidence because as I have written I have slowly begun to talk to people about my writing which in turn has started the conversation around what I am writing and so I have started talking to people about Menopause and what it entails and do you know. I was right, people don't talk about this subject, there are so many people walking around suffering in silence that shouldn't be.

This week I have come across 2 ladies that have started to highlight menopause but mainly connected to exercise which as we know is important but actually is just one small part of the puzzle.

So I would ask that if you are going through this, if anything in this book resonates with you then please start talking, share the book, tell people about it.

Let's together spread the word and support each other with this delight that every single one of us women is going to experience during our life time, everyone one of us, and we are many!

CHAPTER 22

REFERENCES

These are all the accounts/pages/books/podcasts that I have either referenced or found useful on my journey

Instagram Accounts

> @tallyrye
>
> @lucysheridan
>
> @rhitrition
>
> @pandorapaloma
>
> @adrienelouise
>
> @mrshinchhome
>
> @lucymountain
>
> @aliceliveing
>
> @pixienutrition
>
> @amanda.thebe (superb menopause account)
>
> @thesarahpowell

Facebook Pages

> Train Happy Facebook Group
> The Menopause Beauty Tribe
> Amanda Thebe - Fit n' Chips (Superb menopause page)

Literature

    Nourishing Menopause - Margie King

    The Comparison Cure - Lucy Sheridan

    Intuitive Living - Pandora Paloma

    Is Butter a Carb? - Rose Saunt and Helen West

    Just Eat It - Laura Thomas

    Thin side Out - Josie Spinardi

    Intuitive Eating - Evelyn Tribole

    Intuitive Eating - Becky Bellucci

    Health at Every Size - Linda Bacon

    The Happiness Project - Gretchen Rubin

Podcasts

    Fit and Fearless

    Nutrition Matters

    The whey Box

    Wobble

The above may not all be Menopause related but they are what I have used throughout my journey of discovery so I have included them as you might also find them useful. This is just the tip of the iceberg, there are mammoth amounts of self help books out there. This list, like my book, is just a good place to start.

CHAPTER 23

AFTER THOUGHT

So in these pages is just my experiences but as with all these things Menopausal there are others, everyday I hear new things or have new things happen to me.

Hopefully now you have read my book , you will feel a little more normal, you have a little more knowledge and you are ready to get out there and live your life to the full. After all we only get one and why should a small thing like Menopause stop us from being the best versions of ourselves we can possible be!

I am sure that I will continue to learn new things but I hope hand on heart that by sharing this journey of mine I might have helped you just a little. A the very least I have made you laugh and laughter is a great medicine for whatever ails you.

I would like to Thank you all for taking the time to read my journey, if it has helped you then please tell your friends shout it from the rooftops, lets get this information out there for all women.

Good Luck with your journeys

Kim

X

ABOUT THE AUTHOR

Kim Mcintyre

Kim lives currently in North Cyprus but is orignally from West Sussex, England.
This is Kim's first book and a subject matter that she is passionate about.

I hope you have enjoyed reading my book and it has given you some hope. If you have please share it with you friends so we can get the word out, so we can all feel a little more normal.

I would love it if you could leave a review, this is another way that we can spread the message together.

Thank you x

Printed in Great Britain
by Amazon

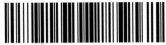